Printed in the United Kingdom.

First Printing, 2016

ISBN 13: 978-1-84481-002-4

ISBN 10: 1-84481-002-X

**Warning and Disclaimer**

# Hero's Journey
## 2016

## N. Rey | darebee.com

# Thank you!

Thank you for purchasing *Pocket Workouts*, DAREBEE project print edition. DAREBEE is a non-profit global fitness resource dedicated to making fitness accessible for everyone, no matter the circumstances. The project is supported exclusively via user donations and paperback royalties.

After printing cost and store fees every book developed by DAREBEE project makes $1 and it goes directly into our project maintenance and development fund.

Each sale helps us keep the DAREBEE resource growing, maintain it and keep it up. Thank you for making a difference in its future!

# Introduction

Hero's Journey is a role-play fitness program inspired by every hero's transformation from minion to master. Each day takes you through a stage of the journey, presents you with fresh challenges, opportunities and threats. Each of these is accompanied by exercises that test your skill, push your performance and require you to adapt and develop in order to go on.

The role play scenario transports your mind into situations where you face incredible odds and have to fight to survive. In the process you get to change not just physically but also mentally. The routines are designed to immerse you into imaginative scenarios where you have to push your mind, forcing yourself to dig deep to find the willpower to not give up, fight the good fight and come out the other side.

The journey is 60 days long and it is totally transformative. When you have really traveled the hero's path and have gone through your quest, you will have shed uncertainty, fear and doubt along with excess body weight. You will have forged a new character out of yourself, build strength and endurance and developed power. You will stand confident in who you are and what you can do: a true hero to yourself.

Only check Karma when you see Hero's Journey - Karma symbol
or on days: 2, 9, 11, 15, 18, 23, 31, 33, 42 & 60. Try not to check ahead.

# Instructions

### Reps (repetitions) per exercise
Reps are usually located next to each exercise's name. Number of reps is always a total number for both legs / arms / sides. It's easier to count this way: e.g. if it says 20 climbers, it means that both legs are already counted in - it is 10 reps each leg.

*Reps to failure* means to muscle failure = your personal maximum, you repeat the move until you can't. It can be anything from one rep to twenty, normally applies to more challenging exercises. The goal is to do as many as you possibly can.

*Reps throughout the day* means that your goal is to get all of the numbers in by the end of the day. You can split the total number of reps for the day into manageable sets. In some of the challenges it is a necessity, in others an optional extra. Using this option will help you complete any challenge on your fitness level. Ideally, you want to do as fewer sets as possible. Most of the time you will begin to need this option a week or two into the challenge.

### Levels & Difficulty
Each workout has three levels of difficulty: I, II and III. If you are new to exercise or you haven't done any training in a long while you should start on Level I. You don't have to stay on level I consistently, if you feel that you can do more, you can advance a level. Level III is the hardest level of difficulty and it can be pretty challenging to complete. Think of it as game levels of difficulty.

### Rest between sets
There is no rest between exercises - only after sets, unless specified otherwise.

*Up to 2 minutes rest* means you can rest for up to 2 minutes but the sooner you can go again the better. Eventually your recovery time will improve naturally, you won't need all two minutes to recover - and that will also be an indication of your improving fitness.

**Before you start:** Look over the workout you chose to do and make sure you understand all of the exercises illustrated so it doesn't slow you down once you have started.

**Video Exercise Library  http://darebee.com/exercises**

# Modifications / Exercise Alternatives

If you are recovering from an injury, have a mild disability that prevents you from doing certain moves, have bad knees or are suffering from back pain and you want to avoid high impact exercises but you still want to stay active and try some of the workouts from this book, try these modifications.

The modifications will also be suitable if you are trying to keep the noise you make to a minimum – it's handy if you live in an apartment and your neighbours are ... not very understanding people.

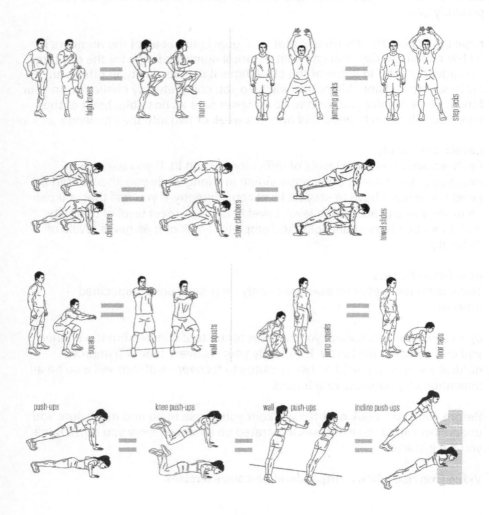

## Notes & Points

# HERO'S JOURNEY

© darebee.com

**Day 1** | Press "START" to play

**LEVEL I** 60 reps
**LEVEL II** 100 reps
**LEVEL III** 200 reps

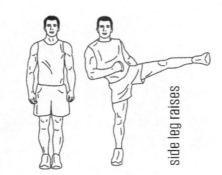

side leg raises

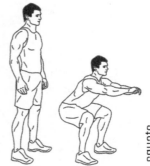

squats

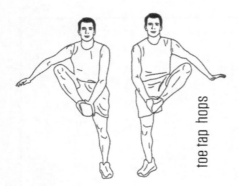

toe tap hops

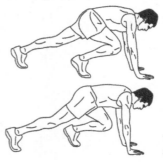

climbers

Complete all in one go or split into manageable sets.
Take as much time as you need.

## Notes & Points

# HERO'S JOURNEY

**Day 2** | Stranger at the crossroads

**LEVEL I** 5 sets
**LEVEL II** 7 sets
**LEVEL III** 10 sets

2 minutes rest between sets

---

**OPTION A** MIND YOUR OWN BUSINESS

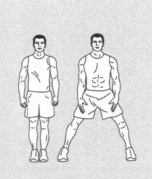

**60** half jacks

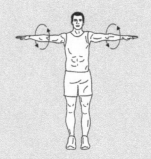

**40** raised arm circles

**OPTION B** GET INVOLVED

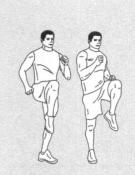

**60** high knees

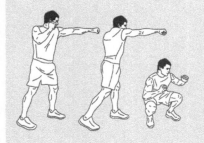

**20 combo**
jab + jab + cross + squat

## Notes & Points

# HERO'S JOURNEY
© darebee.com

**Pick a weapon(s) for your quest.
Your choice will influence
character development.**

Each item represents additional training and will represent it from here on.
See charts for each item and training reference for each **weapons' practice** day.

### heavy sword
pull-ups
upper body strength
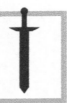

### hammer
free weights
upper body strength

### bow and arrow
running
speed, agility & endurance

### lasso
jump rope
speed, agility & endurance
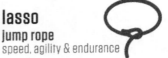

### ribbon
martial arts
extra fighting practise

### magic ring
elbow planks
rock hard core

### Body Armor
wrist weights minimum 0.5 kg / 1 lb
ankle weight minimum 1kg / 2 lb
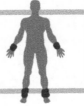

You can proceed without an item but you will still have to try at least one on for the day.

## Notes & Points

# HERO'S JOURNEY
© darebee.com

**Day 4** | Under the stars

No time to rest for the wicked.
You may not be  totally wicked
but even your stops have to train
your body for the journey ahead.

**PART 1**  **8 reps each** | **3 sets** | 2 minutes rest between sets

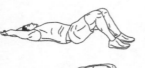
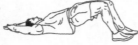

bridges

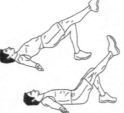

one legged bridges

flutter kicks

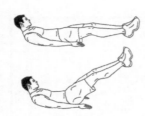

leg raises

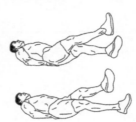

scissors

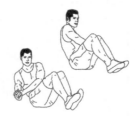

sitting twists

**PART 2**

superman stretches
**10 reps each** | **3 sets**
60 seconds rest between sets

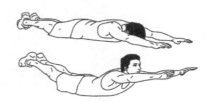

## Notes & Points

# HERO'S JOURNEY

**Day 5** | Journey Through The Woods

**LEVEL I**   5 sets
**LEVEL II**  7 sets
**LEVEL III** 10 sets

2 minutes rest between sets

The woods are thick and hard to get through. The path has to be created from scratch. The strength of your legs has to serve you well, here.

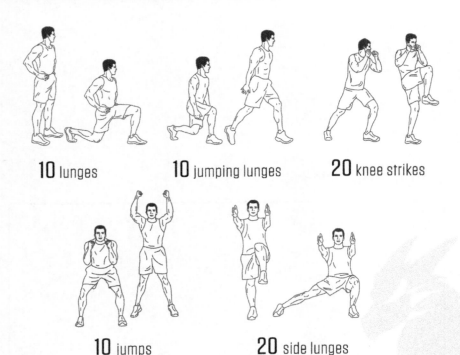

**10** lunges          **10** jumping lunges          **20** knee strikes

**10** jumps          **20** side lunges

**You find a dragon egg. Keep the egg YES / NO ?**

If you keep the egg, a baby dragon will hatch and become your side kick.
A side kicks fights with you, giving you an additional (optional) minute
of recovery between each set.

## Notes & Points

# HERO'S JOURNEY
© darebee.com

**Day 6** | Blocked path

**The road ahead is blocked.
Your upper body strength will help you
push through.**

---

**PART 1**    **LEVEL I** 5 sets   **LEVEL II** 7 sets   **LEVEL III** 10 sets
2 minutes rest between sets

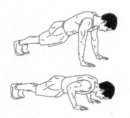 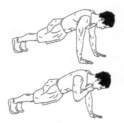 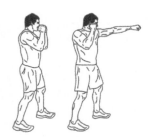

**to failure** push-ups     **10** shoulder taps     **20** punches

---

**PART 2**   **Weapons' Practice**

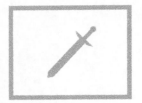  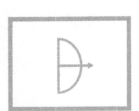

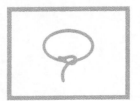 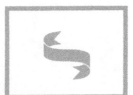 

## Notes & Points

# HERO'S JOURNEY

© darebee.com

**Day 7** | The Oracle

**LEVEL I** 5 sets
**LEVEL II** 7 sets
**LEVEL III** 10 sets

2 minutes rest between sets

YOU ARE NOT AND WILL NEVER BE A HERO.

Prove him wrong.
No one can to tell you
who you can or cannot be.

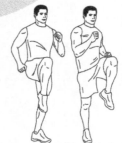

**20** high knees

**2** plank jump-ins

**20** high knees

**2** plank jump-ins

**20** high knees

**2** plank jump-ins

**20** high knees

**2** plank jump-ins

**20** high knees

**2** plank jump-ins

BONUS QUEST add a **push-up**  after each high knees exercise

## Notes & Points

# HERO'S JOURNEY

© darebee.com

**Day 8** | **A Night to Remember**

Your rest time
is your charge-up time.
Power up the core.

## PART 1    10 reps each | 3 sets | 2 minutes rest between sets

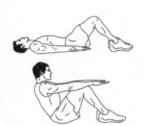

sit-ups

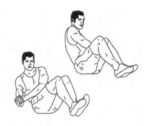

sitting twists

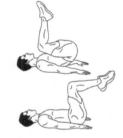

reverse crunches

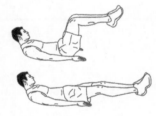

crunch kicks

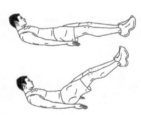

leg raises

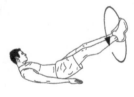

raised leg circles

## PART 2

superman stretches
**10 reps each** | **3 sets**
60 seconds rest between sets

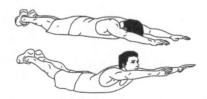

## Notes & Points

# HERO'S JOURNEY

**Day 9** | Collapsing Bridge

The ground is falling under you. You need to be strong to survive.

---

## CLEAR THE BRIDGE.

### 12 reps each

**LEVEL I** 5 sets
**LEVEL II** 7 sets
**LEVEL III** 10 sets
2 minutes rest between sets

toe tap hops

side-to-side jumps

climbers

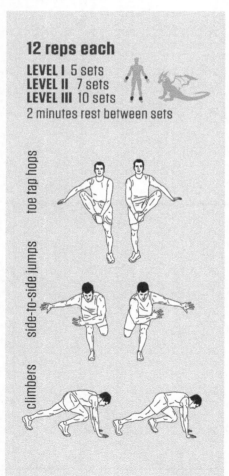

## CLEAR THE BRIDGE WITH A SINGLE JUMP.

# 200
**jump squats**

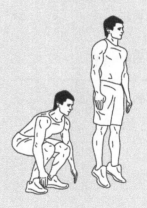

in one go
short breaks
( under 20 seconds )
are ok

## Notes & Points

# HERO'S JOURNEY

© darebee.com

**Day 10** | Into the Storm

**The elements are against you. Fight back.**

---

**PART 1** — **LEVEL I** 5 sets  **LEVEL II** 7 sets  **LEVEL III** 10 sets
2 minutes rest between sets

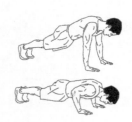 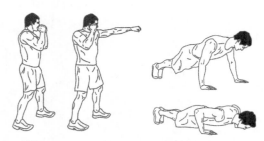

**to failure** push-ups          **40** punches          **to failure** wide grip push-ups

---

**PART 2**  **Weapons' Practice**

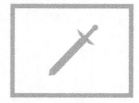  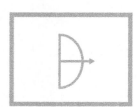

 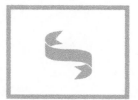 

## Notes & Points

# HERO'S JOURNEY

© darebee.com

**Day 11** | **Close Call**

**You have been badly wounded in the storm. How badly?**

| Iamgonnadie | It's bad but not _that_ bad | 'Tis but a scratch |
|---|---|---|
| **5 sets** | **7 sets** | **10 sets** |
| 10 knee strikes | 10 high knees | 10 high knees |
| 10 step jacks | 10 half jacks | 10 jumping jacks |
| 10 side leg raises | 10 squats | 10 jump squats |
| 20 knee strikes | 20 high knees | 20 high knees |
| 20 step jacks | 20 half jacks | 20 jumping jacks |
| 20 side leg raises | 20 squats | 20 jump squats |

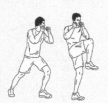
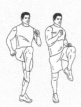
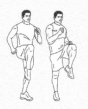

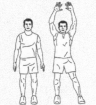

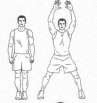

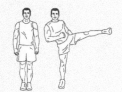
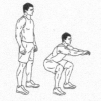
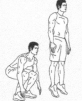

## Notes & Points

# HERO'S JOURNEY

© darebee.com

## Day 12 | Refuge

Someone found you unconscious
and is tending to your wounds.
Take it easy, you will need your strength
soon enough.

Hold each pose for **10 seconds**
or **count** to **10** and repeat
the sequence again
focusing on the other side.

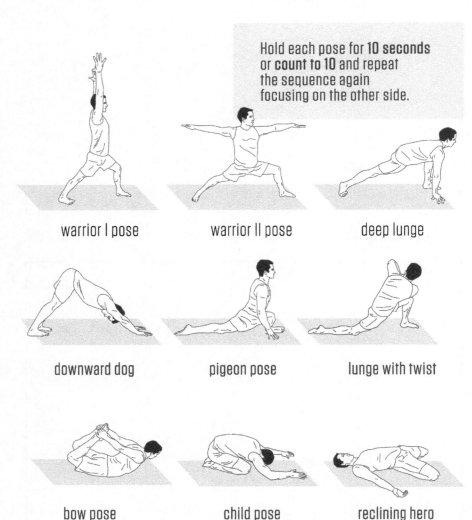

warrior I pose

warrior II pose

deep lunge

downward dog

pigeon pose

lunge with twist

bow pose

child pose

reclining hero

## Notes & Points

# HERO'S JOURNEY

© darebee.com

**Day 13** | New Bonds

You wake up in a new place.
No one has attacked you... yet.

---

**PART 1**   **LEVEL I** 5 sets   **LEVEL II** 7 sets   **LEVEL III** 10 sets
2 minutes rest between sets

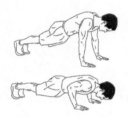

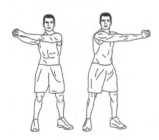

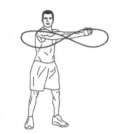

**to failure** push-ups          **20** side chops          **20** infinity chops

"draw" ∞ symbol in the air

---

**PART 2**   **Weapons' Practice**

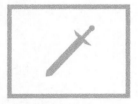

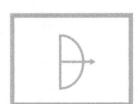

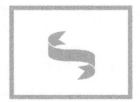

## Notes & Points

# HERO'S JOURNEY

© darebee.com

**Day 14** | ...and you are cornered

**LEVEL I**   30 combos each fight
**LEVEL II**   50 combos each fight
**LEVEL III**   100 combos each fight

3 fights in total | non-stop

## You are surrounded by enemies. Defend yourself!

**FIGHT (1)**

jab
jab
cross
squat

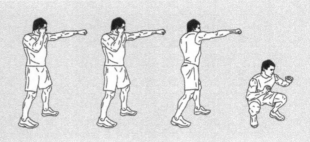

**FIGHT (2)**

backfist
side kick

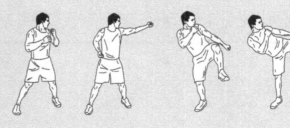

**FIGHT (3)**

knee strike
elbow strike

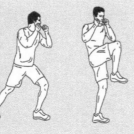 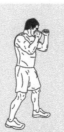 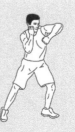

## Notes & Points

# HERO'S JOURNEY

© darebee.com

**Enemy dragons attack.
Fight for the innocent,
protect the weak!**

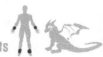

1 bar = 1 set
2 minutes rest between sets

▰ ▰ ▰ ▰ ▰ ▰ ▰ ▰ ▰ ▰ ▰ ▰

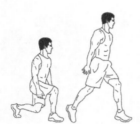

**10** jumping lunges

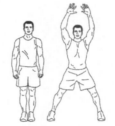

**10** jumping jacks

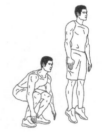

**10** jump squats

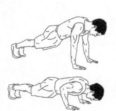

**to failure** push-ups

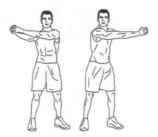

**20** side chops

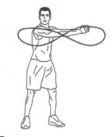

**20** infinity chops

**ROAR! the moment you complete your last set.
Record and post it online #hearmeroar**

## Notes & Points

# HERO'S JOURNEY

© darebee.com

**Day 16** | **The sun goes down**

**Earn your rest by preparing for the new day.**

---

**PART 1** | **12 reps each** | **3 sets** | 2 minutes rest between sets

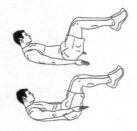

hundreds

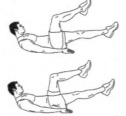

air bike crunches

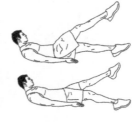

flutter kicks

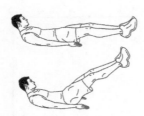

leg raises

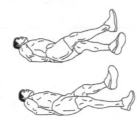

scissors

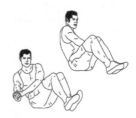

sitting twists

---

**PART 2**

superman stretches
**10 reps each** | **3 sets**
60 seconds rest between sets

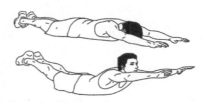

## Notes & Points

# HERO'S JOURNEY

© darebee.com

**Day 17** | Double Trouble

**Trouble never comes in single doses.
Dig deep to survive.**

---

**PART 1**  **LEVEL I** 5 sets  **LEVEL II** 7 sets  **LEVEL III** 10 sets
2 minutes rest between sets

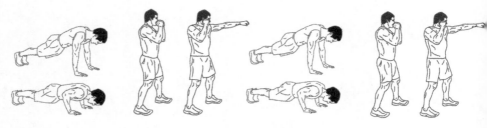

**to failure** push-ups    **20** punches    **to failure** push-ups    **20** punches

---

**PART 2**  **Weapons' Practice**

 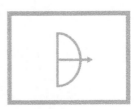
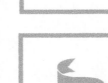
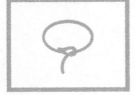 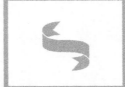 

## Notes & Points

# HERO'S JOURNEY

© darebee.com

**Day 18** | The Chase

**catch one** 5 sets
**catch two** 7 sets
**catch 'em all** 10 sets

2 minutes rest between sets

They are getting away!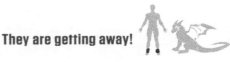

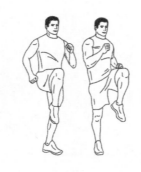

20 high knees
6 climbers
20 high knees
6 climbers
20 high knees
6 climbers

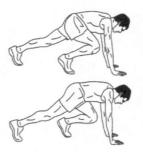

20 high knees
6 climbers
20 high knees
6 climbers

**BONUS QUEST**    add a **push-up**  after each high knees exercise

## Notes & Points

# HERO'S JOURNEY

© darebee.com

**Day 19** | Ambush

The enemy has surprised you.
Do not get taken without a fight.

**LEVEL I** 5 sets **LEVEL II** 7 sets **LEVEL III** 10 sets
2 minutes rest between sets

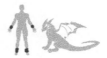

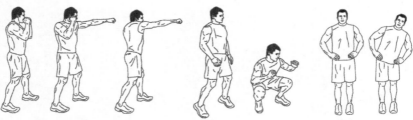

**20 combos** jab + jab +cross          **10** squat + side bend

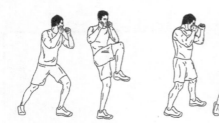

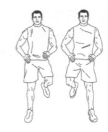

**20 combos** knee strike + elbow strike          **10** side-to-side hops

OPTIONAL SUBQUEST

**1000 punches**
Inflict some serious damage
before you are captured

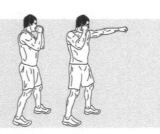

## Notes & Points

# HERO'S JOURNEY

© darebee.com

**Day 20** | Escape

**Set yourself free.
Your hands are tied behind your back.**

**PART 1**    **20 reps each** | **5 sets** | 2 minutes rest between sets

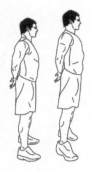

calf raises

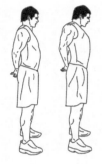

back stretches

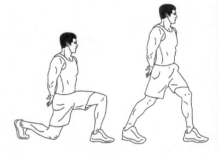

split lunges

**PART 2**

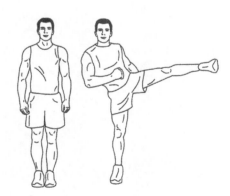

**side leg raises**
**LEVEL I**    200 reps
**LEVEL II**   300 reps
**LEVEL III**  400 reps
reps throughout the day

**BONUS QUEST**    Perform side leg raises with hands (tied) behind your back

## Notes & Points

# HERO'S JOURNEY

© darebee.com

**Day 21** | The Return

**Your quest continues
and so does your training.**

---

**PART 1**  **LEVEL I** 5 sets  **LEVEL II** 7 sets  **LEVEL III** 10 sets
2 minutes rest between sets

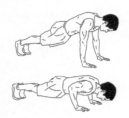
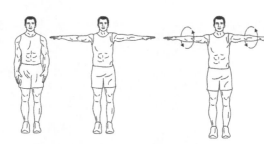

**to failure** push-ups          **40** arm raises          **40** raised arm circles

---

**PART 2**  **Weapons' Practice**

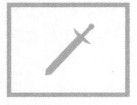

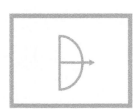

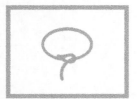
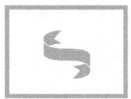

## Notes & Points

# HERO'S JOURNEY

**Day 22** | Allies

**Prove yourself worthy of the allegiance of others.**

**LEVEL I** 5 sets  **LEVEL II** 7 sets  **LEVEL III** 10 sets
2 minutes rest between sets

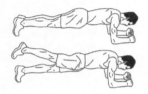

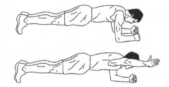

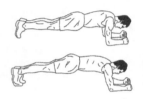

**10** plank leg raises    **10** plank arm raises    **10** body saw

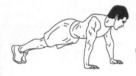

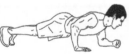

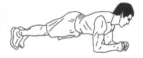

**10** up and down planks

OPTIONAL SUBQUEST

**2000 punches**
Inflict some serious damage
before you are captured

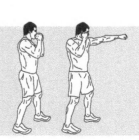

## Notes & Points

# HERO'S JOURNEY
© darebee.com

**got away**  3 sets
**got away, wounded**  4 sets
**caught**  5 sets

2 minutes rest between sets

Catch the spy before he gets away.
Go as fast as possible.
Go for 60 seconds flat out.

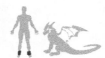

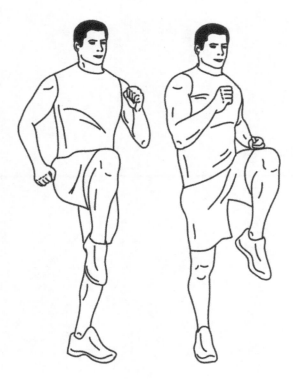

SUB QUEST        hit a total of **90 high knees** in 60 seconds

## Notes & Points

# HERO'S JOURNEY

© darebee.com

**Day 24** | Core Power

Increase your chances of survival
by strengthening your core.
Make the arrows bounce off our abs.

**PART 1** | **14 reps each** | **3 sets** | 2 minutes rest between sets

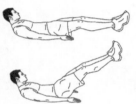

leg raises

pulse ups

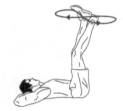

infinity circles

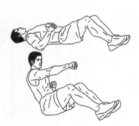

sit-up punches

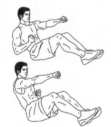

sitting punches

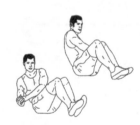

sitting twists

## PART 2

superman stretches
**10 reps each** | **3 sets**
60 seconds rest between sets

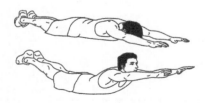

## Notes & Points

# HERO'S JOURNEY

© darebee.com

**Day 25** | Down to business

**Weapons need strength.
Wield yours more powerfully.**

---

**PART 1**    **LEVEL I** 5 sets   **LEVEL II** 7 sets   **LEVEL III** 10 sets
2 minutes rest between sets

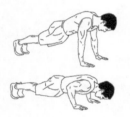 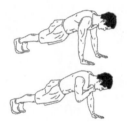 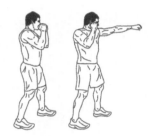

**to failure** push-ups     **20** shoulder taps     **40** punches

---

**PART 2**   **Weapons' Practice**

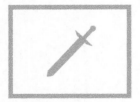  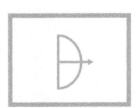

 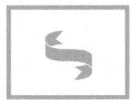 

## Notes & Points

# HERO'S JOURNEY

**Day 26** | Warrior Spirit

**Level I**   3 sets
**Level II**   4 sets
**Level III**   5 sets

2 minutes rest between sets

**True warriors never give up. Endure.**

**5** burpees
ten second rest
**5** burpees
ten second rest
**10** burpees
ten second rest
**5** burpees
ten second rest
**5** burpees

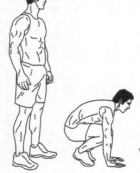
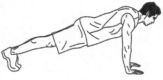

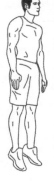

**Tip**   count to 10 for the ten second rest

## Notes & Points

# HERO'S JOURNEY

**Day 27** | Seven Assassins

Defeat all seven.
60 seconds rest
between each fight.

## — EACH FIGHT —

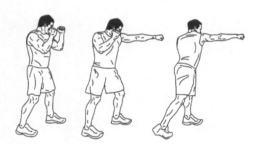

**40combos** jab + jab + cross

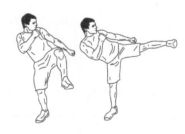

**40** side kicks

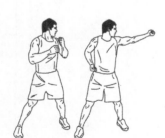

**20** backfists

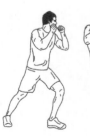

**20** knee strikes

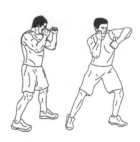

**20** elbow strikes

## Notes & Points

# HERO'S JOURNEY
© darebee.com

**Day 28** | Under the stars

No time to rest for the wicked.
You may not be totally wicked
but even your stops have to train
your body for the journey ahead.

**PART 1** | **14 reps each** | **3 sets** | 2 minutes rest between sets

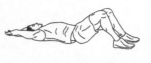
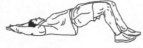

bridges

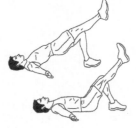

one legged bridges

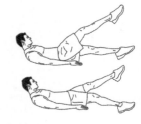

flutter kicks

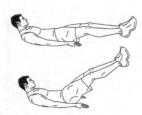

leg raises

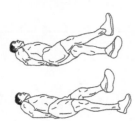

scissors

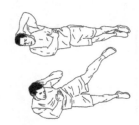

side knifejacks

**PART 2**

superman stretches
**10 reps each** | **3 sets**
60 seconds rest between sets

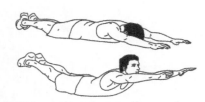

## Notes & Points

# HERO'S JOURNEY

© darebee.com

**Day 29** | Power Within

**Look inside yourself
for the strength to go on.**

**PART 1**  **LEVEL I** 5 sets  **LEVEL II** 7 sets  **LEVEL III** 10 sets
2 minutes rest between sets

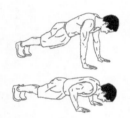 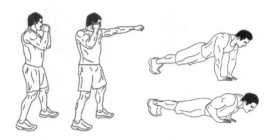

**to failure** push-ups        **40** punches        **to failure** close grip push-ups

**PART 2**  **Weapons' Practice**

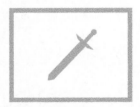  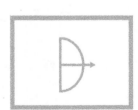

 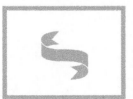 

## Notes & Points

# HERO'S JOURNEY

© darebee.com

**Heroism is endurance
for one moment more.**

## plank

repeat 3 times during the day

**LEVEL I**   30 seconds
**LEVEL II**  2 minutes
**LEVEL III** 3 minutes

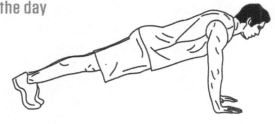

## wall-sit

repeat 3 times during the day

**LEVEL I**   30 seconds
**LEVEL II**  2 minutes
**LEVEL III** 3 minutes

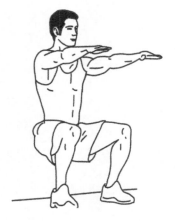

## Notes & Points

# HERO'S JOURNEY

© darebee.com

**Day 31** | The Town Burns

**How many people can you save?**

| 40% saved | 60% saved | 80% saved |
| --- | --- | --- |
| **5 sets** | **7 sets** | **10 sets** |
| 20 high knees | 20 high knees | 20 high knees |
| 20 squats | 20 squats | 20 jump squats |
| 20 shoulder taps | 20 push-ups | 20 push-ups |

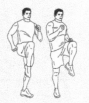 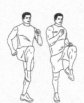 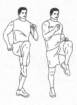

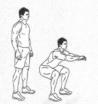 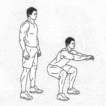 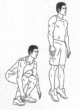

 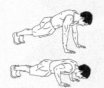 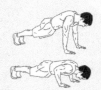

## Notes & Points

# HERO'S JOURNEY

**Day 32** | Aftermath

**Recover from the disaster.
Find the strength to go on.**

**PART 1**  **3 sets** | 60 seconds rest between sets

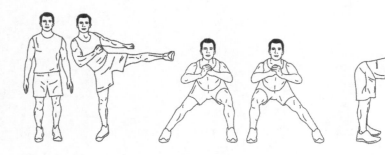

**20** side leg raises  **10** side-to-side lunges  **20** deadlifts

**PART 2**

## 3 minutes

raised arm hold

Stand up and raise your arms
in front of you shoulder length height
and hold them there
for 3 minutes.

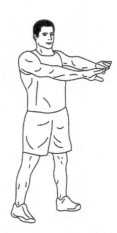

## Notes & Points

# HERO'S JOURNEY

**Day 33** | Journey to the Mountain

**A higher destiny awaits you
but first, you must get there.**

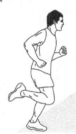

## PART 1

**10,000**
steps walk
8 km or 5 miles

LEVEL I    80 push-ups
LEVEL II   100 push-ups
LEVEL III  150 push-ups

throughout the day

# OR

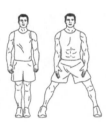

LEVEL I   5 sets
LEVEL II   7 sets
LEVEL III  10 sets
REST up to 2 minutes

50 half jacks
5 push-ups
50 half jacks
5 push-ups
50 half jacks
5 push-ups

## PART 2  Weapons' Practice

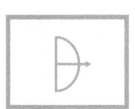

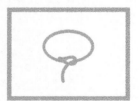

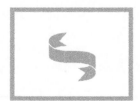

## Notes & Points

# HERO'S JOURNEY

**Day 34** | The Climb

**Giving up is not an option.**

**LEVEL I** 400 slow climbers
**LEVEL II** 600 slow climbers
**LEVEL III** 800 slow climbers

split the total reps
into manageable sets

*It is not the mountain
we conquer
but ourselves.*

## Notes & Points

# HERO'S JOURNEY

© darebee.com

**Day 35** | The Trials

**The guru at the top of the mountain gives you three trials.**

## PART 1

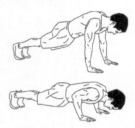
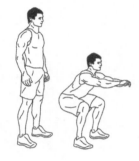
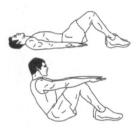

**First Trial**
**3 sets** to failure
push-ups

30 seconds
rest between sets

**Second Trial**
**3 sets** to failure
squats

30 seconds
rest between sets

**Third Trial**
**3 sets** to failure
sit-ups

30 seconds
rest between sets

## PART 2

**3 sets** to failure
wall-sit

30 seconds
rest between sets

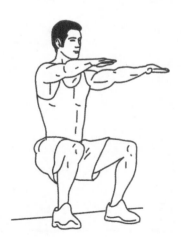

## Notes & Points

# HERO'S JOURNEY

© darebee.com

**Day 36**
**Peace on top of the mountain**

---

**PART 1**  Early morning, pre-breakfast routine **21 reps each**

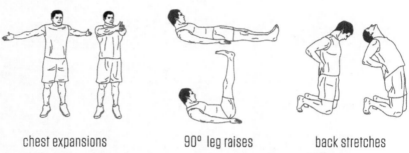

chest expansions          90° leg raises          back stretches

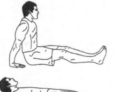
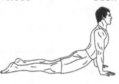
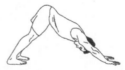

table stretch          upward dog stretch

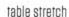

**PART 2**

**10 Minute Meditation**
Sit down, close your eyes, relax.

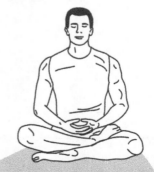

## Notes & Points

# HERO'S JOURNEY

© darebee.com

**Day 37** | Lesson #1  Strength

**True strength comes from muscle control.**

**PART 1**

**LEVEL I** 5 sets  **LEVEL II** 7 sets  **LEVEL III** 10 sets
**LEVEL I** 4 reps  **LEVEL II** 6 reps  **LEVEL III** 8 reps
up to 60 seconds rest between sets
Perform each exercise as slowly as possible.
Example: count to 10 as you lower yourself to the floor
and count to 10 as you come up - that's one rep.

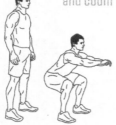

squat

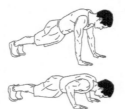

push-up

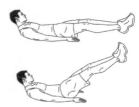

leg raises

**PART 2**  **Weapons' Practice**

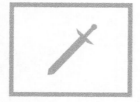

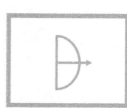

## Notes & Points

# HERO'S JOURNEY

Day 38 | Lesson #2  Speed

**Speed makes you harder to fight, difficult to beat.**

**LEVEL I** 5 sets  **LEVEL II** 7 sets  **LEVEL III** 10 sets
60 seconds rest between sets
Perform each exercise asfast as you can.

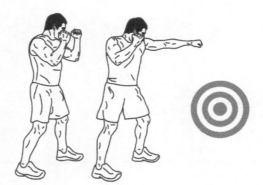

**30 seconds**
= 60 punches
in total

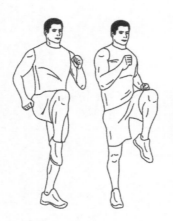

**30 seconds**
= 90 high knees
in total

## Notes & Points

# HERO'S JOURNEY

© darebee.com

**Day 39** | Lesson #3 Control

**Control makes you
more precise.**

---

## PART 1

**LEVEL I** 5 sets  **LEVEL II** 7 sets **LEVEL III** 10 sets
60 seconds rest between sets | keep your arms up between #2 and #3

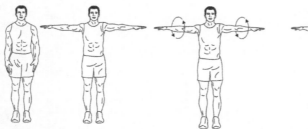
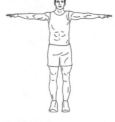

**60** arm raises          **60** raised arm circles          **20-count** raised arm hold

---

## PART 2

## 20 minutes non-stop movement

e.g., punches, kicks, half jacks, hop on the spot, push-ups,
high knees, crunches, arm raises **no breaks**

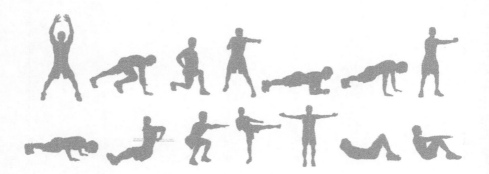

## Notes & Points

# HERO'S JOURNEY

© darebee.com

**Day 40** | Time to move on

**You've learned all there is here. Time to move on.**

**PART 1** | **18 reps each** | **3 sets** | 2 minutes rest between sets

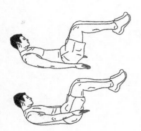

hundreds

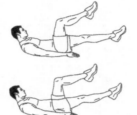

air bike crunches

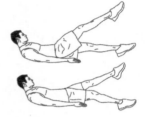

flutter kicks

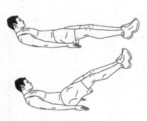

leg raises

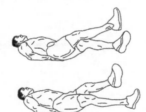

scissors

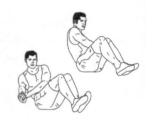

sitting twists

**PART 2** | **blindfold**
stand on one leg, arms out
to sides – then close your eyes
(or use blindfold)

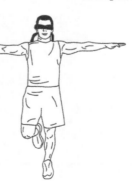

**60 seconds**

## Notes & Points

# HERO'S JOURNEY

© darebee.com

**Day 41** | The Return. Take Two.

**And you are back again.
Your quest continues
and so does your training.**

**LEVEL I** 5 sets  **LEVEL II** 7 sets  **LEVEL III** 10 sets
2 minutes rest between sets

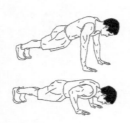
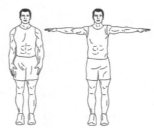
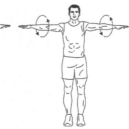

**to failure** push-ups      **50** arm raises      **50** raised arm circles

**PART 2**   **Weapons' Practice**

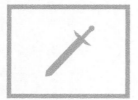

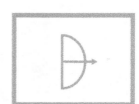
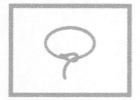

## Notes & Points

# HERO'S JOURNEY

© darebee.com

**Be clever or be strong. Fight, either way**

**LEVEL I** 5 sets
**LEVEL II** 7 sets
**LEVEL III** 10 sets

2 minutes rest between sets

## OPTION A   ATTACK HEAD ON

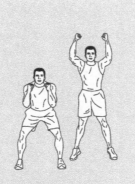

**60** jumps

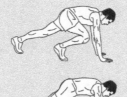

**40** climbers

## OPTION B   SPLIT THE FORCES

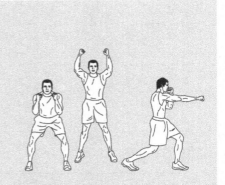

**40** jump cross punches

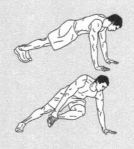

**20** climber taps

## Notes & Points

# HERO'S JOURNEY

© darebee.com

**Day 43** | The Betrayal

Nothing ever goes according to plan.

Step 1 ) Go through the sequence as fast as you can.
Step 2) Pass out.

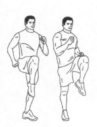

**100** high knees

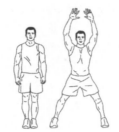

**90** jumping jacks

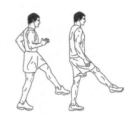

**80** straigh leg bounds

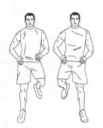

**70** side-to-side hops

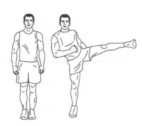

**60** side leg raises

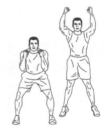

**50** jumps

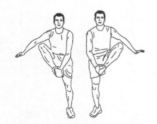

**40** toe tap hops

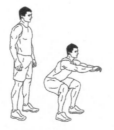

**30** squats

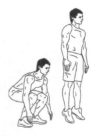

**20** jump squats

## Notes & Points

<br>

# HERO'S JOURNEY

© darebee.com

**Day 44** | Bed Rest & Recovery

**20 reps each** | **3 sets**
60 seconds rest between sets

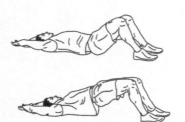

bridges

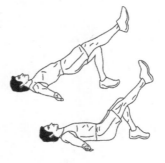

one legged bridges

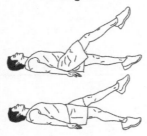

flutter kicks

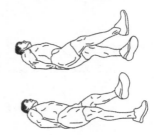

scissors

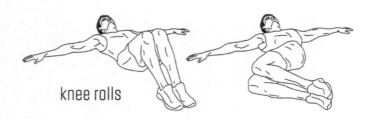

knee rolls

## Notes & Points

# HERO'S JOURNEY

© darebee.com

**Day 45** | Getting Stronger

**Level up
and face your enemies.**

**PART 1**  **LEVEL I** 5 sets  **LEVEL II** 7 sets  **LEVEL III** 10 sets
2 minutes rest between sets

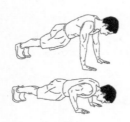 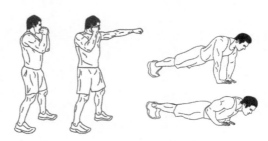

**to failure** push-ups          **60** punches          **to failure** close grip push-ups

**PART 2**  **Weapons' Practice**

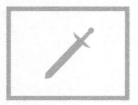  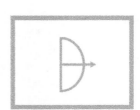

 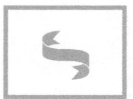 

## Notes & Points

# HERO'S JOURNEY
© darebee.com

**Level I** 3 sets
**Level II** 4 sets
**Level III** 5 sets

2 minutes rest between sets

**Build your speed
and become formidable.
Go for 60 seconds flat out.**

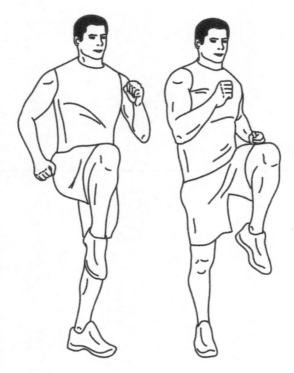

SUB QUEST    hit a total of **120 high knees** in 60 seconds

## Notes & Points

# HERO'S JOURNEY

**Day 47** | Ultimate Control

**Level I** 5 sets
**Level II** 7 sets
**Level III** 10 sets

2 minutes rest between sets

**Achieve control over who you are. Keep your arms up at all times**

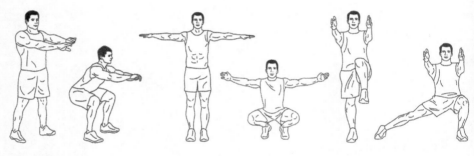

**10** squats          **10** sumo squats          **10** side lunges

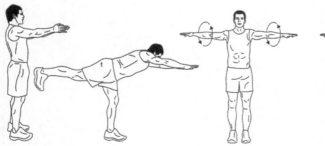
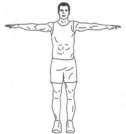

**10** balance stretch          **10** raised arm circles          **10-count** arm hold

## Notes & Points

# HERO'S JOURNEY

© darebee.com

**Day 48** | Under the stars

**The final batle approaches.
Every day counts now.**

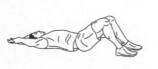

bridges

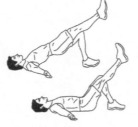

one legged bridges

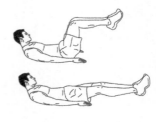

crunch kicks

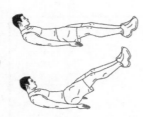

leg raises

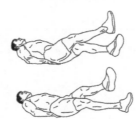

scissors

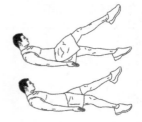

flutter kicks

**PART 2**

superman stretches
**10 reps each**  |  **3 sets**
60 seconds rest between sets

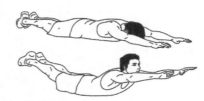

## Notes & Points

# HERO'S JOURNEY

© darebee.com

**Day 49** | Power Up

Go past every limit.
Know no boundary.

---

**PART 1**  **LEVEL I** 5 sets  **LEVEL II** 7 sets  **LEVEL III** 10 sets
2 minutes rest between sets

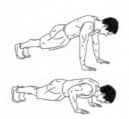
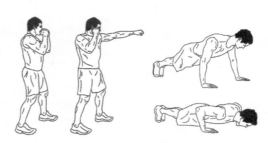

**to failure** push-ups          **60** punches          **to failure** wide grip push-ups

---

**PART 2**  **Weapons' Practice**

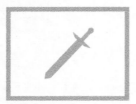

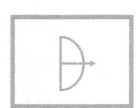

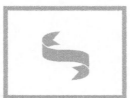

## Notes & Points

# HERO'S JOURNEY

© darebee.com

**Pull everything you know together.**

**LEVEL I** 5 sets  **LEVEL II** 7 sets  **LEVEL III** 10 sets
2 minutes rest between sets

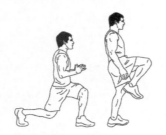

**20** step-ups

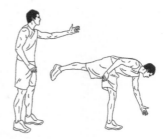

**20** single leg bends

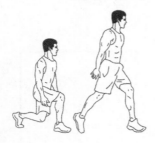

**10** jumping lunges

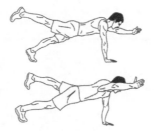

**10** alt arm / leg raises

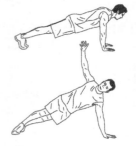

**10** plank rotations

OPTIONAL SUBQUEST

## 3000 punches

Inflict some serious damage before you are captured

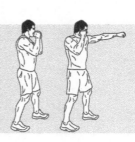

## Notes & Points

# HERO'S JOURNEY

© darebee.com

**Day 51** | Final Transformation

**Let the true hero be born inside yourself.**

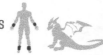

**PART 1**  **LEVEL I** 5 sets  **LEVEL II** 7 sets  **LEVEL III** 10 sets
60 seconds rest between sets

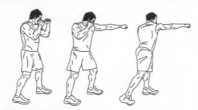
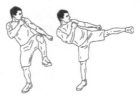

**60combos** jab + jab + cross          **60** side kicks

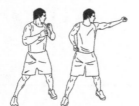
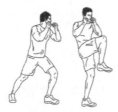
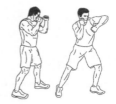

**40** backfists          **40** knee strikes          **40** elbow strikes

**PART 2**  **20 minutes** non-stop movement
e.g., punches, kicks, half jacks, hop on the spot, push-ups,
high knees, crunches, arm raises **no breaks**

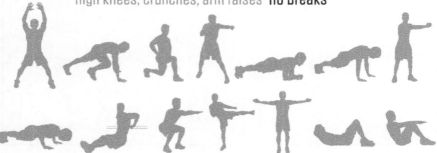

## Notes & Points

# HERO'S JOURNEY

© darebee.com

**Day 52** | **Balance**

**Find your inner balance.**

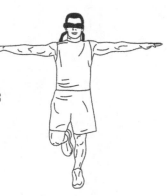

**PART 1** ### blindfold
stand on one leg, arms out
to sides – then close your eyes
(or use blindfold)

## 60 seconds

**PART 2** | **10 reps each** | **3 sets** | 60 seconds rest between sets

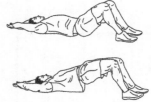

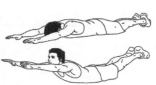

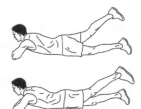

bridges          superman stretches          reverse flutter kicks

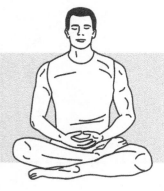

OPTIONAL SUBQUEST

## 10 Minute Meditation
Sit down, close your eyes, relax.

## Notes & Points

# HERO'S JOURNEY

© darebee.com

**Day 53** | The Final Test

**Your upper body strength will help you push through.**

---

**PART 1**   **LEVEL I** 5 sets  **LEVEL II** 7 sets  **LEVEL III** 10 sets
2 minutes rest between sets  -  Hands never off the floor

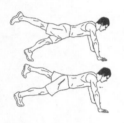 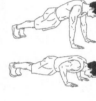 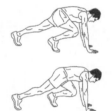 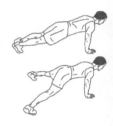

**10** plank leg raises    **to failure** push-ups    **10** climbers    **10** plank jacks

**PART 2**   **Weapons' Practice**

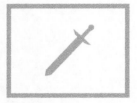  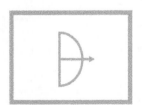

 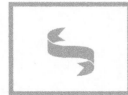 

## Notes & Points

# HERO'S
# JOURNEY

**Day 54** | The Final Skill "Stealth"

**Be silent. Be deadly.**

© darebee.com

---

**PART 1**   **LEVEL I** 5 sets  **LEVEL II** 7 sets  **LEVEL III** 10 sets
2 minutes rest between sets    -   Don't make a sound.

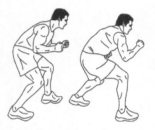

**20steps** half squat walk

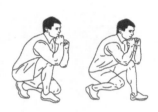

**20steps** duck walk

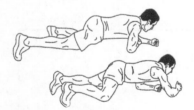

**20** army crawl

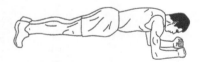

**20-count** elbow plank

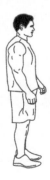

**PART 2**   **20 minutes** of Pure Stealth
Stay still for 20 minutes.

## Notes & Points

# HERO'S JOURNEY
© darebee.com

**Day 55** | The Final Challenge "100"
**A true hero never gives up.**

**100 reps** in total each exercise | split into manageable sets
**Level I** throughout the day **Level II** repeat once **Level III** twice in one day

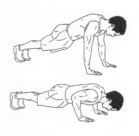

push-ups

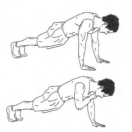

shoulder taps

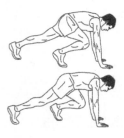

climbers

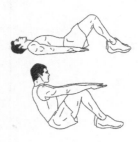

sit-ups

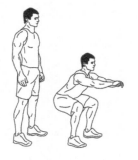

squats

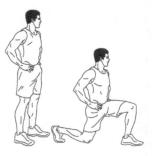

lunges

## Notes & Points

# HERO'S JOURNEY
© darebee.com

**Day 56** | The Awakening

Hold each pose for 20 seconds
(count to 20 ) and repeat the routine
again focusing on the other side.

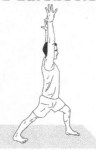
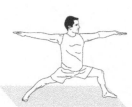
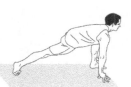

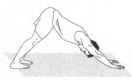
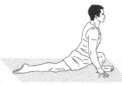
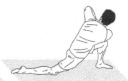

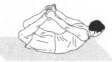
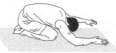
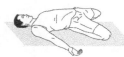

## 10 Minute Meditation
Sit down, close your eyes, relax.

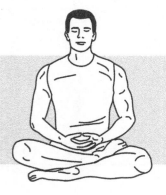

## Notes & Points

# HERO'S JOURNEY

© darebee.com

**PART 1**

**LEVEL I** 5 sets  **LEVEL II** 7 sets  **LEVEL III** 10 sets   whole combo = 1 se
**LEVEL I** 60 reps  **LEVEL II** 80 reps  **LEVEL III** 100 reps
2 minutes rest between sets

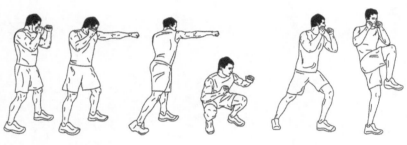

jab + jab + cross          squat          knee strike

**PART 2**   **Weapons' Practice**

 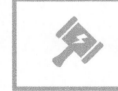 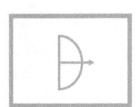

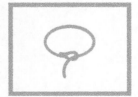 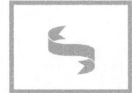 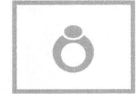

## Notes & Points

# HERO'S JOURNEY

© darebee.com

**LEVEL I** 5 sets  **LEVEL II** 7 sets  **LEVEL III** 10 sets
2 minutes rest between sets

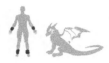

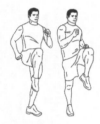

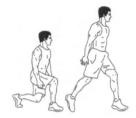

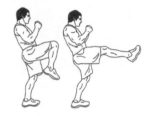

**20** high knees        **20** jumping lunges        **40** front kicks

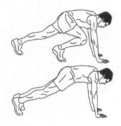

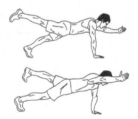

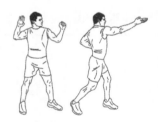

**20** slow climbers     **20** alt arm / leg raises  **20** knife hand strikes

OPTIONAL SUBQUEST

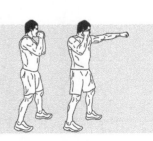

## 3,000 punches
Inflict some serious damage
before you are captured

## Notes & Points

# HERO'S JOURNEY

© darebee.com

**Day 59** | Bodyguard Fight

**Strip the Boss of his protection.**

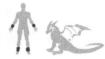

**LEVEL I** 5 sets **LEVEL II** 7 sets **LEVEL III** 10 sets
2 minutes rest between sets

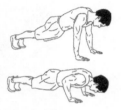

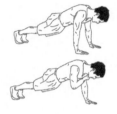

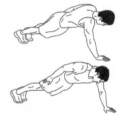

**to failure** push-ups

**20** shoulder taps

**20** thigh taps

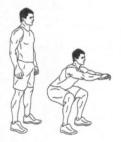

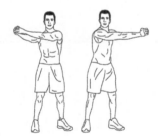

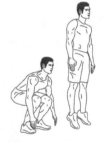

**20** squats

**20** side chops

**20** jump squats

OPTIONAL SUBQUEST

**400 Side Kicks**
Inflict extra damage

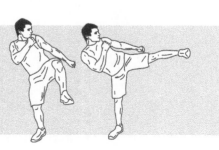

## Notes & Points

# HERO'S JOURNEY

© darebee.com

**Day 60** | Boss Fight

Polish your armor and braid your hair. You are ready. You have been training for this moment. Charge ahead and give it your all!

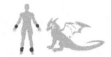

1 bar = 1 set
2 minutes rest between sets

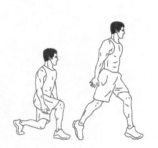

**20** jumping lunges

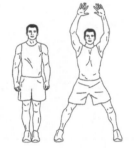

**40** jumping jacks

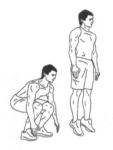

**20** jump squats

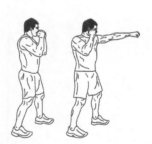

**40** punches

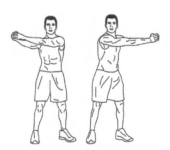

**40** side chops

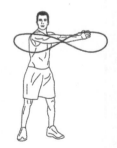

**20** infinity chops

# HERO'S JOURNEY

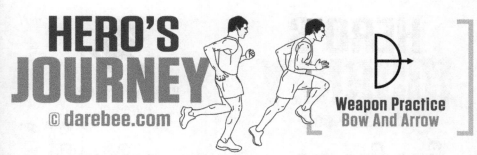

© darebee.com

**Weapon Practice**
**Bow And Arrow**

Train yourself to successfully scout the territory. You will need speed as well as endurance.

| | | | | |
|---|---|---|---|---|
| **DAY 3** | **DAY 6** | **DAY 10** | **DAY 13** | **DAY 17** |
| Map of the Land | 1 minute walk | Endurance | 1 minute run | **20 minutes** |
| | 30 second sprint | | 1 minute rest | walk, jog or run |
| **30 minutes in total** | 1 minute walk | **60 minutes in total** | 5 sets in total | |
| run, jog, walk cycle or row | 30 second sprint | run, jog, walk cycle or row throughout the day | | **10 second sprints** |
| | 1 minute walk | | | 5 sprints in total |
| | 1 minute sprint | | | 2 minute rest between sprints |
| | 5 sets in total | | | |

| | | | | |
|---|---|---|---|---|
| **DAY 21** | **DAY 25** | **DAY 29** | **DAY 33** | **DAY 37** |
| From A to B & back | Endurance | | **20 minutes** | Endurance |
| 50 meters + touchdown | | | walk, jog or run | |
| **5 sprints non-stop** | **60 minutes in total** | 20 second walk | | **60 minutes in total** |
| up to 2 minutes rest | run, jog, walk cycle or row throughout the day | 20 second run | **10 second sprints** | run, jog, walk cycle or row throughout the day |
| **10 sprints non-stop** | | **20 second sprint** | 5 sprints in total | |
| up to 2 minutes rest | | 5 sets in total | 2 minute rest between sprints | |
| **5 sprints non-stop** | | | | |

| | | | | |
|---|---|---|---|---|
| **DAY 41** | **DAY 45** | **DAY 49** | **DAY 53** | **DAY 57** |
| Scout the Territory | | Endurance | **20 minutes** | From A to B & back |
| | | | walk, jog or run | 50 meters + touchdown |
| **30 minutes in total** | 20 second walk | **60 minutes in total** | | **5 sprints non-stop** |
| run, jog, walk cycle or row | 20 second run | run, jog, walk cycle or row throughout the day | **10 second sprints** | up to 2 minutes rest |
| | **20 second sprint** | | 5 sprints in total | **10 sprints non-stop** |
| | 5 sets in total | | 2 minute rest between sprints | up to 2 minutes rest |
| | | | | **5 sprints non-stop** |

# HERO'S
# JOURNEY
## © darebee.com

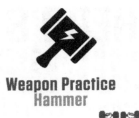

**Weapon Practice**
**Hammer**

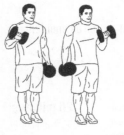

*alternating bicep curls*

 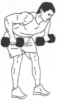

*bent over rows*

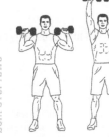

*shoulder press*

Perform each exercise slowly minding your form, keep your core tight. Take 2 full minutes rest after each exercise and each set. All reps are given in total e.g., 10 biceps curls = 5 each arm.

| DAY 3 | DAY 6 ✳ | DAY 10 | DAY 13 | DAY 17 ✳ |
|---|---|---|---|---|
| 8 bicep curls | 40 bicep curls | 8 bicep curls | 8 bicep curls | 50 bicep curls |
| 5 bent over rows | 20 bent over rows | 5 bent over rows | 5 bent over rows | 30 bent over rows |
| 5 shoulder press | 20 shoulder press | 5 shoulder press | 5 shoulder press | 30 shoulder press |
| 3 sets of each | in total for the day | 3 sets of each | 3 sets of each | in total for the day |

| DAY 21 | DAY 25 ✳ | DAY 29 | DAY 33 | DAY 37 ✳ |
|---|---|---|---|---|
| 10 bicep curls | 60 bicep curls | 10 bicep curls | 10 bicep curls | 60 bicep curls |
| 6 bent over rows | 40 bent over rows | 6 bent over rows | 6 bent over rows | 40 bent over rows |
| 6 shoulder press | 40 shoulder press | 6 shoulder press | 6 shoulder press | 40 shoulder press |
| 3 sets of each | in total for the day | 3 sets of each | 3 sets of each | in total for the day |

| DAY 41 | DAY 45 ✳ | DAY 49 | DAY 53 | DAY 57 ✳ |
|---|---|---|---|---|
| 12 bicep curls | 70 bicep curls | 12 bicep curls | 12 bicep curls | 80 bicep curls |
| 8 bent over rows | 50 bent over rows | 8 bent over rows | 8 bent over rows | 60 bent over rows |
| 8 shoulder press | 50 shoulder press | 8 shoulder press | 8 shoulder press | 60 shoulder press |
| 3 sets of each | in total for the day | 3 sets of each | 3 sets of each | in total for the day |

Pick the kind of free weights you can do 8 reps with.
Continue to increase the weight as it gets easier.

✳ use lighter dumbbells

# HERO'S JOURNEY

© darebee.com

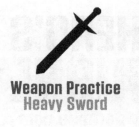

**Weapon Practice
Heavy Sword**

Take as much time to recover between sets as you need Alternatively to pull-ups: you can do negative pull-ups or chin-ups. Chin-ups will focus more on your biceps rather than back.

| | |
|---|---|
| Day 3 | 3 sets pull-ups to failure |
| Day 6 | 10 pull-ups in total for the day |
| Day 10 | 3 sets pull-ups to failure |
| Day 13 | 3 sets pull-ups to failure |
| Day 17 | 15 pull-ups in total for the day |
| Day 21 | 4 sets pull-ups to failure |
| Day 25 | 4 sets pull-ups to failure |
| Day 29 | 20 pull-ups in total for the day |
| Day 33 | 4 sets pull-ups to failure |
| Day 37 | 4 sets pull-ups to failure |
| Day 41 | 25 pull-ups in total for the day |
| Day 45 | 5 sets pull-ups to failure |
| Day 49 | 5 sets pull-ups to failure |
| Day 53 | 30 pull-ups in total for the day |
| Day 57 | 5 sets pull-ups to failure |

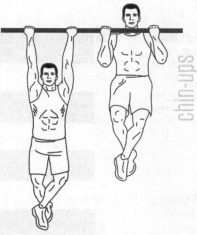

chin-ups

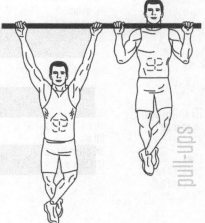

pull-ups

# HERO'S JOURNEY

© darebee.com

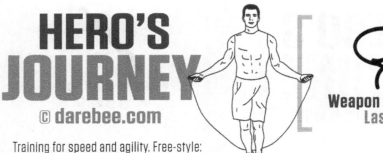

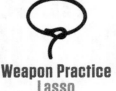

**Weapon Practice
Lasso**

Training for speed and agility. Free-style:
You can vary styles or stick to one.

### DAY 3

**5 minutes**
jump rope
any rest time

FINISH
10 lasso twists
3 sets in total
2 min rest

### DAY 6

60 skips
30 second rest
60 skips
30 second rest
60 skips
2 min rest
5 sets in total

### DAY 10

**10 minutes**
jump rope

in total
throughout
the day

### DAY 13

30 skips
30 second rest
60 skips
30 second rest
120 skips
2 min rest
5 sets in total

### DAY 17

1 min skips
1 min rest
5 sets in total

FINISH
10 lasso twists
3 sets in total
2 min rest

### DAY 21

**10 minutes**
jump rope

in total
throughout
the day

### DAY 25

60 skips
30 second rest
60 skips
30 second rest
60 skips
2 min rest
5 sets in total

### DAY 29

**5 minutes**
jump rope
any rest time

FINISH
15 lasso twists
3 sets in total
2 min rest

### DAY 33

30 skips
30 second rest
60 skips
30 second rest
120 skips
2 min rest
5 sets in total

### DAY 37

1 min skips
1 min rest
5 sets in total

FINISH
20 lasso twists
3 sets in total
2 min rest

### DAY 41

**10 minutes**
jump rope
any rest time

FINISH
25 lasso twists
3 sets in total
2 min rest

### DAY 45

30 skips
30 second rest
60 skips
30 second rest
120 skips
2 min rest
5 sets in total

### DAY 49

1 min skips
1 min rest
5 sets in total

FINISH
30 lasso twists
3 sets in total
2 min rest

### DAY 53

**10 minutes**
jump rope

in total
throughout
the day

### DAY 57

60 skips
30 second rest
60 skips
30 second rest
60 skips
2 min rest
5 sets in total

# HERO'S JOURNEY

## © darebee.com

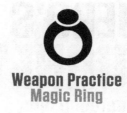

**Weapon Practice**
**Magic Ring**

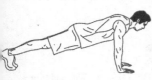
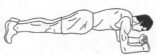
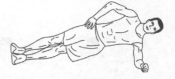

Turn yourself invisible by blending with the environment. Sometimes it's stealth that can save your life.

| DAY 3 | DAY 6 | DAY 10 | DAY 13 | DAY 17 |
|---|---|---|---|---|
| 20 sec plank<br>20 sec elbow plank<br>20 sec side plank<br>2 minute rest<br>3 sets in total | **5 minutes**<br>plank or elbow plank<br>in total<br>throughout the day | 60 sec plank<br>2 minute rest<br>60 sec elbow plank<br>2 minute rest<br>60 sec plank<br>done | **2 minutes**<br>plank<br>or elbow plank<br>3 times in total<br>during the day | 30 sec plank<br>30 sec elbow plank<br>60 sec side plank<br>2 minute rest<br>3 sets in total |

| DAY 21 | DAY 25 | DAY 29 | DAY 33 | DAY 37 |
|---|---|---|---|---|
| **5 minutes**<br>plank or elbow plank<br>in total<br>throughout the day | 60 sec elbow plank<br>2 min side plank<br>2 minute rest<br>3 sets in total | **2 minutes**<br>plank<br>or elbow plank<br>3 times in total<br>during the day | 60 sec plank<br>2 minute rest<br>60 sec elbow plank<br>2 minute rest<br>60 sec plank<br>done | **3 minutes**<br>plank<br>or elbow plank<br>2 times in total<br>during the day |

| DAY 41 | DAY 45 | DAY 49 | DAY 53 | DAY 57 |
|---|---|---|---|---|
| 30 sec plank<br>30 sec elbow plank<br>60 sec side plank<br>2 minute rest<br>3 sets in total | 60 sec elbow plank<br>2 min side plank<br>2 minute rest<br>3 sets in total | **3 minutes**<br>plank<br>or elbow plank<br>2 times in total<br>during the day | **5 minutes**<br>plank or elbow plank<br>in total<br>throughout the day | 60 sec plank<br>2 minute rest<br>60 sec elbow plank<br>2 minute rest<br>60 sec plank<br>done |

# HERO'S JOURNEY

© darebee.com

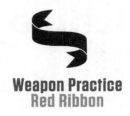
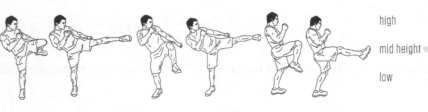

high —

mid height —

low —

Be more than "Enough". Turn your own body into a weapon.

| | | | | |
|---|---|---|---|---|
| **DAY 3** | **DAY 6** | **DAY 10** | **DAY 13** | **DAY 17** |
| 100 turning kicks<br>100 side kicks<br>100 front snap kicks<br>in total for the day | 40 slow side kicks<br>60 sec rest (optional)<br>40 fast side kicks<br>2 minutes rest<br>5 sets in total | **100**<br>double turning kicks<br>low / mid<br>in total for the day | 40 front snap kicks<br>switch leg<br>40 front snap kicks<br>2 minutes rest<br>5 sets in total | 20 turning kicks<br>20 side kicks<br>20 front snap kicks<br>2 minute rest<br>10 sets in total |
| **DAY 21** | **DAY 25** | **DAY 29** | **DAY 33** | **DAY 37** |
| **100**<br>double side kicks<br>low / mid<br>in total for the day | 20 turning kicks<br>20 side kicks<br>20 front snap kicks<br>2 minute rest<br>10 sets in total | 100 turning kicks<br>100 side kicks<br>100 front snap kicks<br>in total for the day | 60 slow side kicks<br>60 sec rest (optional)<br>60 fast side kicks<br>2 minutes rest<br>5 sets in total | **100**<br>double turning kicks<br>low / mid<br>in total for the day |
| **DAY 41** | **DAY 45** | **DAY 49** | **DAY 53** | **DAY 57** |
| 20 turning kicks<br>20 side kicks<br>20 front snap kicks<br>2 minute rest<br>10 sets in total | 80 slow side kicks<br>60 sec rest (optional)<br>80 fast side kicks<br>2 minutes rest<br>5 sets in total | **100**<br>double turning kicks<br>low / mid<br>in total for the day | 40 front snap kicks<br>switch side<br>40 front snap kicks<br>2 minutes rest<br>5 sets in total | 100 turning kicks<br>100 side kicks<br>100 front snap kicks<br>in total for the day |

# HERO'S JOURNEY

© darebee.com

Use the chart below to work out how many points you have earned.

| DAY 1 | I +100  II +200  III +300 |
| DAY 2 | I +100  II +200  III +300 |
| DAY 3 | See the weapons' charts |
| DAY 4 | Part 1 +100   Part 2 +50 |
| DAY 5 | I +100  II +200  III +300 |
| DAY 6 | I +100  II +200  III +300  (WP) |
| DAY 7 | I +100  II +200  III +300  BQ +100 |
| DAY 8 | Part 1 +100   Part 2 +50 |
| DAY 9 | I +100  II +200  III +300  JUMP +300 |
| DAY 10 | I +100  II +200  III +300  (WP) |
| DAY 11 | I +100  II +200  III +300 |
| DAY 12 | +100 points |
| DAY 13 | I +100  II +200  III +300  (WP) |
| DAY 14 | I +100  II +200  III +300 |
| DAY 15 | +50 points per charge |

| DAY 16 | Part 1 +100   Part 2 +50 |
| DAY 17 | I +100  II +200  III +300  (WP) |
| DAY 18 | I +100  II +200  III +300  BQ +100 |
| DAY 19 | I +100  II +200  III +300  OS +200 |
| DAY 20 | P 1 +100  P 2 I +50  II +100  III +150 BQ +50 |
| DAY 21 | I +100  II +200  III +300  (WP) |
| DAY 22 | I +100  II +200  III +300  OS +200 |
| DAY 23 | I +100  II +200  III +300  BQ +200 |
| DAY 24 | Part 1 +100   Part 2 +50 |
| DAY 25 | I +100  II +200  III +300  (WP) |
| DAY 26 | I +100  II +200  III +300 |
| DAY 27 | +100 per assassin ( 700 for all seven ) |
| DAY 28 | Part 1 +100   Part 2 +50 |
| DAY 29 | I +100  II +200  III +300  (WP) |
| DAY 30 | I +50  II +100  III +150 <br> I +50  II +100  III +150 |

I = Level I    II = Level II    III = Level III    OS - optional subquest    BQ - bonus quest    (WP) weapons practice

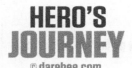

# HERO'S
# JOURNEY
© darebee.com

Use the chart below to work out how many points you have earned.

| | |
|---|---|
| **DAY 31** | I +100  II +200  III +300 |
| **DAY 32** | Part 1 +100  Part 2 +100 |
| **DAY 33** | I +100  II +200  III +300  (WP) |
| **DAY 34** | I +100  II +200  III +300 |
| **DAY 35** | Part 1 +200  Part 2 +100 |
| **DAY 36** | Part 1 +100  Part 2 +50 |
| **DAY 37** | I +100  II +200  III +300  (WP) |
| **DAY 38** | I +100  II +200  III +300 |
| **DAY 39** | P1 I +100  II +200  III +300  P2 +200 |
| **DAY 40** | Part 1 +100  Part 2 +50 |
| **DAY 41** | I +100  II +200  III +300  (WP) |
| **DAY 42** | I +100  II +200  III +300 |
| **DAY 43** | +300 points |
| **DAY 44** | +100 points |
| **DAY 45** | I +100  II +200  III +300  (WP) |

| | |
|---|---|
| **DAY 46** | I +100  II +200  III +300  BQ +200 |
| **DAY 47** | I +100  II +200  III +300 |
| **DAY 48** | Part 1 +100  Part 2 +50 |
| **DAY 49** | I +100  II +200  III +300  (WP) |
| **DAY 50** | I +100  II +200  III +300  OS +400 |
| **DAY 51** | P1 I +100  II +200  III +300  P2 +200 |
| **DAY 52** | Part 1 +100  Part 2 +50  OS +50 |
| **DAY 53** | I +100  II +200  III +300  (WP) |
| **DAY 54** | P1 I +100  II +200  III +300  P2 +200 |
| **DAY 55** | I +100  II +200  III +300 |
| **DAY 56** | +100 points  OS +50 |
| **DAY 57** | I +100  II +200  III +300  (WP) |
| **DAY 58** | I +100  II +200  III +300  OS +400 |
| **DAY 59** | I +100  II +200  III +300  OS +400 |
| **DAY 60** | +100 points for every set completed |

I = Level I   II = Level II   III = Level III   OS - optional subquest   BQ - bonus quest   (WP) weapons practice

1 PULL-UP +20
1 CHIN-UP +10
1 NEGATIVE PULL-UP +5

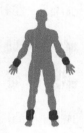

**+ 50**

for every day
you wear
the armor

| DAY 3 | + 50 |
| DAY 6 | + 100 |
| DAY 10 | + 50 |
| DAY 13 | + 50 |
| DAY 17 | + 100 |
| DAY 21 | + 50 |
| DAY 25 | + 150 |
| DAY 29 | + 50 |
| DAY 33 | + 50 |
| DAY 37 | + 150 |
| DAY 41 | + 50 |
| DAY 45 | + 200 |
| DAY 49 | + 50 |
| DAY 53 | + 50 |
| DAY 57 | + 200 |

| DAY 3 | + 200 |
| DAY 6 | + 100 |
| DAY 10 | + 400 |
| DAY 13 | + 100 |
| DAY 17 | + 300 |
| DAY 21 | + 200 |
| DAY 25 | + 400 |
| DAY 29 | + 100 |
| DAY 33 | + 300 |
| DAY 37 | + 400 |
| DAY 41 | + 200 |
| DAY 45 | + 100 |
| DAY 49 | + 400 |
| DAY 53 | + 300 |
| DAY 57 | + 200 |

| DAY 3 | +100 LT +50 | | DAY 3 | +50 | | DAY 3 | +100 |
| DAY 6 | +200 | | DAY 6 | +100 | | DAY 6 | +100 |
| DAY 10 | +300 | | DAY 10 | +50 | | DAY 10 | +100 |
| DAY 13 | +200 | | DAY 13 | +50 | | DAY 13 | +200 |
| DAY 17 | +100 LT +50 | | DAY 17 | +100 | | DAY 17 | +200 |
| DAY 21 | +300 | | DAY 21 | +50 | | DAY 21 | +100 |
| DAY 25 | +200 | | DAY 25 | +300 | | DAY 25 | +100 |
| DAY 29 | +100 LT +50 | | DAY 29 | +300 | | DAY 29 | +200 |
| DAY 33 | +200 | | DAY 33 | +300 | | DAY 33 | +100 |
| DAY 37 | +100 LT +50 | | DAY 37 | +200 | | DAY 37 | +200 |
| DAY 41 | +100 LT +50 | | DAY 41 | +300 | | DAY 41 | +200 |
| DAY 45 | +200 | | DAY 45 | +400 | | DAY 45 | +100 |
| DAY 49 | +100 LT +50 | | DAY 49 | +200 | | DAY 49 | +200 |
| DAY 53 | +300 | | DAY 53 | +300 | | DAY 53 | +100 |
| DAY 57 | +200 | | DAY 57 | +300 | | DAY 57 | +100 |

There is no choice without consequence. No action without a karmic effect. You made yours on this journey. Every hero has to live by the effect of the choices made.

# Day 2

You chose to get involved. The stranger you helped helps you back on Day 7 when you meet The Oracle. Do one fewer sets that day (i.e. Level I = 4 sets, Level II = 6 sets, Level III = 9 sets). As an added bonus – the stranger punches the oracle in the face on your behalf.

You chose to mind your own business. You are alone. Add one set to each level on Day 7.

# Day 9

You cleared the bridge with a single jump. You can bask in your awesomeness.

You scrambled and scrambled as it collapsed. You've lost your backpack and with it - your dinner.

# Day 11

Iamgonnadie... but did you die? Celebrate life by doing 200 skips by the end of the day. Skip away, grasshopper.

It was bad, but not that bad. What's that? You are feeling dizzy? Everything is going blank... you lost your sight. It will return in 30 minutes.

It was but a scratch. Your wound still bleeds so you remember of an old family remedy your great grandma packed you before you started your quest. You look through your bad and you find it – it's a slice of pie. Life's good. Enjoy!

# Day 15

You could only master five charges. Take a moment of silence for those who have perished at this day.

Talk to no one for 2 hours.

Your seven charges helped protect the weak but your bravery came at a cost
– your dragon was badly wounded. Your dragon will return to your side only on day 17.

Ten charges make you the people's champion! On day 17, when Double trouble strikes,
reduce each level by 1 set. All hail the Mighty Hero!

## Day 18

You caught one. And the bastard bit you! It looks infected, better take care of it asap.
To avoid infection, don't use that arm (pick one) for the next 2 hours.  Oh yeah and also..... See consequences of "Caught two"
You caught two. Good catch. The one that got away, though, pocketed your bread. Oh well, no bread today.
You caught them all. Congratulations!  After a thorough body search you discover that last one has a chocolate bar on his person. Confiscate it for your own consumption.


## Day 23

The spy got away. Are you serious? Who lets a spy get away? He'll, like, tell stuff to EVERYONE.
And he sure does. Your location has been revealed and now everyone has a description of you and knows your location. You have go into hiding. No phone, no internet, no TV for 2 hours.
The spy got away... but he was wounded. Well, at least you got him good. His injuries (an arrow to the knee)  prevent him from talking (mostly because he can't shut up about the arrow) so your enemies have a somewhat unclear description of you. It's still good to be careful– no internet for an hour, just to be safe.
You caught the sneaky bastard. On his person you found enemy plans and whatnot.
You can now cancel one of the unwanted consequences down the line or drop one of the sets without any consequences or drop one weapons' practice session.


## Day 31

Saved 40%. The town suffered heavy losses. Most of the food supply was burnt.  You will have to ration your food. No dinner today. Or tomorrow.
Saved 60%. The town is saved but some of the food was destroyed. You sadly lose your dinner but overall it's not too bad. I mean, it could have been worse.
Most of the town survived because of you. Congratulations! The grateful townsfolk name the day after you and call it a holiday. Take the day off your chores and celebrate with a nice meal.

## Day 33

The journey to the mountaintop was long and hard. If you chose the 10,000 steps, your shoes just couldn't take the pace. They gave out before you. Spend thirty minutes with your feet up and get someone to massage them for you.

If you chose the sets, while you were busy with them, some dastardly person stole your shoes. Go barefoot for sixty minutes.

## Day 42

You used your brain, not brawn. Splitting the forces allows you to preserve your numbers and gain ground. You have also captured a high ranking officer who has, after some persuasive talking to, revealed a secret weakness of those close to the final boss, their circle of trust has been broken.

On Day 59, against the Bodyguard you can now reduce each level by one set.

Brute force choice. Not everything can be resolved with overwhelming force. You may have won but you suffered heavy losses that have weakened you. You now need to fight harder to win. On Day 59 add an extra 400 punches at the end of the level.

## Day 60

The Boss fight is your toughest challenge yet, but you have been preparing for this.

If you just did five sets or less you just weren't quite ready enough. You need to start from the beginning and make better choices the second time round.

If you did between six and eight sets, it is a draw. It has been a real struggle getting here, but you can take it. Don't give up now. Pick yourself up and fight another day. You have another chance to settle the score.

Nine or ten sets and you have defeated the final BOSS. VICTORY! A legend is born.

# Other Books in the same series

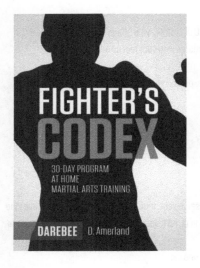

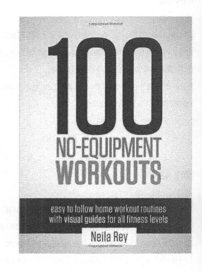

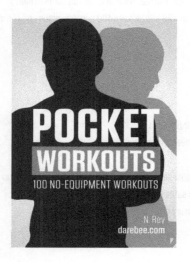

Printed in August 2021
by Rotomail Italia S.p.A., Vignate (MI) - Italy